The Post-menopausal Woman

Leading a healthy life.

Living longer.

By Alex Montgomery

First Edition 2014

Introduction

Post-menopause is the last stage in the menopause phase. The average age for post-menopause is 55.

Post-menopause can be a time of anxiety or can be a time where many women feel liberated. With post-menopause, however, women are at greater risk of heart disease, osteoporosis and cancer.

In order to live longer and enjoy life, women need to lead a healthy life by exercising, eating healthy and practicing good habits.

Post-menopause is a phase in women's lives that can span up to 30 years or more. This is a time that will bring women different opportunities and experiences. It is a time to enjoy.

Disclaimer

Table of Contents

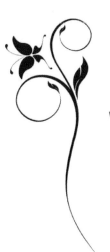

What is Post-menopause

What is Post-menopause

Post-menopause is the last stage of menopause. There are three stages of Menopause: Perimenopause, Menopause and post menopause.

Post-menopause is the time when a woman does not reproduce anymore following menopause (after your last period). Post-menopause begins between the late 40's and early 60's. It is the beginning of the rest of a woman's life.

During this phase women are at greater risk of developing heart disease, osteoporosis, high blood pressure and stroke.

Some women think that all the symptoms associated with perimenopause and menopause will disappear, but that is often not the case. Symptoms are very similar to those during perimenopause.

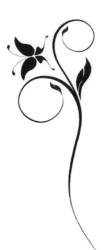

What causes Post-menopause

What causes Post-menopause

Post-menopause can be caused either by hormonal changes or external circumstances.

Hormonal changes

During post-menopause, hormone levels decline and fluctuation in estrogen, testosterones and progesterone might still cause symptoms similar to those experienced during perimenopause, but much less significant. Those symptoms eventually will disappear.

External circumstances

Post-menopause is generally caused by hormonal changes. However, sometimes external circumstances may cause a woman to enter menopause and post-menopause much earlier in her life.

Some of those factors are:

- Smoking and drinking heavily
- Constant period of stress
- Surgery (due to cancer or other health issues)
- Radiation or chemotherapy

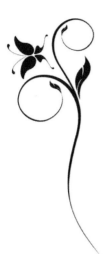

Symptoms during Post-menopause

Symptoms during Post-menopause

Following the menopause transition and menopause, most women stop feeling those uncomfortable symptoms associated with perimenopause. But unfortunately that is not always the case. Hormone changes are still occurring during post-menopause causing symptoms similar to those during perimenopause.

Most women will experience a renewed sense of energy and wellbeing. Others report some remaining symptoms that can continue as long as another 10 years following menopause.

Here are some of the most commons symptoms:

Vaginal dryness: Occurs when estrogen levels decrease causing thinning and shrinking of the vaginal walls. Some women may also experience itching and burning and pain with vaginal sexual activity. Lubricants or vaginal estrogen rings can help increase moisture and sexual enjoyment. You should talk to a health care provider to rule out other medical conditions such as, allergies, skin conditions, foreign bodies, vulvar dystrophies and malignancies.

Vaginal discharge: Is a sign of atrophying vagina. This also can cause vaginal dryness and itching. The discharge is usually thin and may be stained with a trace of blood. While this symptom is not uncommon, if you experience heavy and frequent flow of blood seek medical advice as it might be a more serious condition.

Incontinence: Bladder changes are common during post-menopause as estrogen levels decreases and the pelvic muscles become weaker. Doing pelvic muscle exercises might help to reduce symptoms.

Urinary tract infection (UTI): Estrogen is responsible for keeping the acidity of vaginal fluids making the urinary tract tissue stronger, and making it hard for bacteria to enter the bladder. As women enter post-menopause, estrogen levels diminish, causing bacteria to grow and enter the urinary tract. These bacteria hide in the underlying tissue until they are activated to cause infection. Some UTI's include: urethritis (infection of the urethra), cystitis (bladder infection) and pyelonephritis (kidney infection). You must seek medical attention to treat any UTI's. Early treatment with antibiotics can prevent infection from spreading to the kidneys.

Weight gain: The biggest contributor to increased weight gain during post-menopause is the diminishing levels of estrogen. During post-menopause women can put on up to 10 to 20 pounds without even making changes in their diets. The body naturally tries to retain body fat in order to increase estrogen levels. The metabolism also slows down and lean body fat weight declines. Other factors contributing to weight gain are stress and depression. Postmenopausal women need to increase metabolism by exercising and heating healthy.

Some uncommon symptoms are:

Vaginal bleeding: During post-menopause, heavy bleeding is uncommon. You should seek medical attention as it could be symptoms of some serious health issues such as cancer or some menopause treatments such as hormone replacement therapy.

Hot flashes: are experienced during the menopause transition and are not very common during post-menopause. These symptoms may be experienced from time to time during post-menopause but should be less noticeable. If you experience hot flashes during post-menopause, seek medical advice as it could indicate some other serious disease.

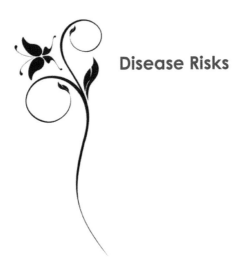

Disease Risks

Disease Risks

Due to the decrease of female hormones during post-menopause, women are at greater risk of: Osteoporosis (thinning of the bones), increase of cardiovascular diseases (high blood pressure, heart attack and stroke) and breast cancer, among others.

Osteoporosis

Osteoporosis is a disease of the bones, where parts of the bone become fragile and susceptible to fracture. When bones lose minerals such as calcium, quicker than the body is able to replace them, the bones lose strength, get less dense and break more easily. This usually occurs among women who have reached menopause, as estrogen is a key hormone to maintain bone strength. Having 30% less bone mass than men, women are more prone to get osteoporosis as they age. It is estimated that women lose up to 10 % of bone mass in the first five years after menopause.

There are two types of osteoporosis:

- Primary: common among women during post-menopause over the age of 70.

- Secondary: affects middle age people, generally caused by medication, chronic illnesses or too much exercise.

Factors that increase the risk of osteoporosis are:

- Decrease of estrogen after menopause
- Family history and body type. Europeans, Asians or people that are "small-boned" are more at risk
- Smoking and excessive drinking
- Lack of exercise
- Lack of calcium
- Low levels of vitamin D
- High intake of caffeine

Symptoms and complications:

- There are no specific symptoms or pain, but there is an increased risk of fracture in the hipbones, wrist or spine.
- Osteoporosis can also cause chronic back pain.

Diagnosis:

Diagnosis is done by using a DEXA (dual energy X-ray absorptiometry) scan that measures bone density.

Measuring bone density will determine the risk of fracture. Having a bone density that is too low will usually conclude that you have osteoporosis.

CT (computerized tomography) can also help to check conditions of the bones.

Reducing risk:

In order to prevent osteoporosis or reduce bone fracture, women during post-menopause should:

- Increase calcium intake and aim to 1200mg daily.
- Increase vitamin D doses if you are over 50, to between 800IU and 2000IU.
- Stop smoking
- Limit alcohol intake
- Reduce excessive caffeine intake
- Exercise (weight bearing exercise and resistance training)

Treatment:

There are many medications to treat osteoporosis or prevent it. You should discuss with your doctor the benefits and risks associated with these medications and your individual requirements in accordance with your age, health issues and your risk of fracture.

- Bisphosphonates
- Selective estrogen receptor modulators
- Calcitonin
- Denosumab
- Testosterone
- Hormone replacement therapies
- Parathyroid hormone
- Vitamin D and calcium supplements

Cardiovascular disease

Women after menopause have a high risk of heart disease. It is one of the main causes of death in postmenopausal women.

Women who smoke, lead a sedentary life, suffer from hypertension, diabetes, high cholesterol, have a history of heart disease or have a poor diet stand a greater risk of having cardiovascular disease.

High blood pressure and hypertension increases in women after menopause due to hormonal changes. Changes in hormones leaves women more sensitive to salt and weight gain contributing to high blood pressure. Aging and the loss of endogenous estrogen production after menopause together with increase in high blood pressure add to the high incidence of hypertension in older women. More than 25% of the female adult world population is hypertensive.

Women with high blood pressure and hypertension have a higher risk of developing fatal heart diseases.

Women with risk of cardiovascular disease should make lifestyle changes that include:

- Eating a diet low in saturated fats and cholesterol
- Eat whole grains and vegetables
- Limit sodium
- Stop smoking
- Maintain a healthy weight
- Exercise most days

Breast cancer

Breast cancer is very common in postmenopausal women. These cancers are hormone receptor positive. As estrogen levels drastically decline during post-menopause, the body makes estrogen in fat tissue, including in the breast tissue fat cells. As women get older, the fat cells in the breast produce a greater amount of enzymes called aromatase, producing more estrogen. This locally produced estrogen appears to trigger breast cancer.

Breast cancer risk can be reduced by medications classified as endocrine therapies to block estrogen production (often used after surgery) or hormone replacement therapy. Both treatments have side effects, but often the benefits outweigh the risks.

You should discuss with the best treatment for you with your doctor if you have been diagnosed with breast cancer or pose a greater risk of getting breast cancer.

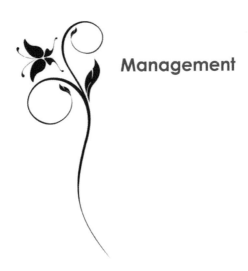

Management

Management

You can better manage post-menopause if you reduce stress, have regular pap tests and breast checks, avoid smoking, have an exercise routine and keep a healthy diet.

Regular Pap test and breast checks are important to have every two years. See your health care provider for more information. Free tests are often offered to women over 40.

Avoid smoking as it is associated with osteoporosis as well as lung cancer and coronary disease.

Reduce stress, some women experience stress due to the hormonal changes. Other factors such as aging parents, children's demands or children living home, career changes or financial issues can add to the stress and intensify the symptoms during post-menopause. Stress can also increase high blood pressure, gastric reflux, headaches, depression or other heart diseases.

You can reduce stress by:

- Exercising
- Eating well
- Avoiding caffeine and alcohol
- Sleeping adequately
- Talking to friends
- Doing breathing exercises
- Yoga and Meditation
- Trying new hobbies
- Pampering yourself
- Having fun
- Seeing a therapist

Regular exercise is important to maintain good health and keep your bones healthy. Exercise produces endorphins that increase your energy and mood. Exercise at least 30-45 minutes most days.

Exercise also helps you to increase your metabolism and reduce weight gain. It is important, however, that you see a doctor first to determine the appropriate exercise for you.

Set realistic goals and start slow. Try to exercise about the same time every day and drink plenty of water.

Avoid high impact activities (reduce risk of fractures), do weight bearing exercises and resistance training exercises (or strength training).

Weight bearing exercises are those carried out by your feet such as walking, dancing, Zumba, running, tennis, biking or jogging. These exercises are great to increase your heart rate, build muscle and burning calories.

Swimming is also another great way to exercise. It is low impact, helps you increase your metabolism and works all your muscles.

Strength training: uses weights such as dumbbells, or machines or other type of weights. It will help you to strengthen the bones, build muscle and burn fat. It will also help you to boost your metabolism. Select weights that can be heavy enough to exercise your muscles in 12 repetitions to begin with.

You can also include exercises that include your own body weight such as push-ups, plank or even yoga.

A healthy diet will help you to reduce symptoms, keep a healthy weight and fight disease. It will also help you to feel more energetic and strengthen your immune system.

During this new phase women should:

Consume enough calcium: As women get closer to menopause and post-menopause, bones become thinner and you can suffer the risk of getting osteoporosis. You need to up your intake of calcium and vitamin D in order to keep your bones strong.

Women under 50 should take up to 1000 mg of calcium per day and 1200 mg after the age of 50. You need to eat and drink at least two servings of dairy product and calcium rich foods, such as dairy products, fish, broccoli and legumes. You may also need some supplements.

Increase iron intake: It is recommended that during this period women allow for 8mg per day by eating three servings of iron rich foods per day. Iron is found in lean meat, fish, eggs, leafy green vegetables, nuts and grain products. You might also need to consume iron tablets.

Boost fiber: Fiber will help you to lose weight and also reduce estrogen during perimenopause. Aim for soluble fiber and eat between 25-35g per day. Fiber can be found in grains like whole wheat bread, quinoa, oatmeal, nuts, barley, lentils, some fruits such as apple or berries and vegetables like spinach.

Drink water: As a general rule drink 8 glasses of water.

Reduce salt and sugar intake: Too much salt can cause high blood pressure. Too much sugar will trigger more hot flashes, besides increasing the risk of heart disease and weight gain.

Eat fruits and vegetables: Fruits and vegetables have many health benefits, providing vitamins, fibers and minerals. During post-menopause fruit and vegetables potentially helps to keep a healthy weight and keep your bones strong. You should include between 1 ½ -2 cups of fruit and 2-3 cups of vegetables per day in your diet.

Consume cruciferous vegetables. Cruciferous vegetables are considered very high in antioxidants, vitamin C, and high in vitamin A carotenoids, folic acid and fiber. They also contain vitamin K which helps with inflammation and cancer prevention. They are, however, well known for their phytonutrients that help the enzymes that improve estrogen metabolism, allowing excess estrogen to leave the body. Some of the cruciferous vegetables are: brussel sprouts, bok choy, broccoli, cauliflower, cabbage, kale, horseradish, radish, watercress, turnip, arugula and mustards greens. These vegetables are best when they are fresh or raw. If they are to be cooked, the best option is to chop them and let them sit for several minutes before cooking. The preferred method of cooking is steamed.

Cut on processed food and high in fat: Limit the amount of fat, saturated fat and processed foods. You should aim for no more that 25% to 30% of fats in your diet with saturated fats being less than 7%. Good fats include foods that are rich in omega 3, found in fish and olive oil. Saturated fat increases cholesterol and the risk of heart diseases. Fat foods are usually high in calories and have little nutrition value. Also limit your intake in trans fatty acids such as margarine, packaged cookies, crackers and vegetable oils. Eat lean meats. Avoid whole milk and ice creams and reduce cheese intake.

Eat proteins: Eat lean meats, fish poultry, eggs and nuts. Eat at least 5 to 6 ounces of meat or equivalent, or 25-35 g per day. Proteins are necessary for muscle synthesis, growth, repair and maintenance of skeletal muscle.

Eat berries: Berries are a great source of antioxidants that help to clean your liver. They also help to improve cardiovascular health, keep blood sugar in control, help eye health, boost metabolism and have many nutritional benefits. Include raspberries, goji berries, strawberries, blackberries, blueberries and cranberries among others in your diet.

Eat food high in phytoestrogen in moderation: Phytoestrogens are naturally found in some foods, imitating the function of estrogen in the body. You should eat these foods in moderation as too much phytoestrogen can cause tissue growth and disturb your endocrine system. Some of the foods that include phytoestrogen are: fruits and vegetables, legumes, peas, beans, bran, wholegrain and flaxseeds.

Eat food rich in vitamin C, complex B vitamins and carotene: Look for food rich in vitamin C such as: cantaloupe, kiwi, tomato, peaches, orange, bananas, artichoke, carrots, corn, cauliflower and lima beans. Include foods rich in carotene such as: kale, spinach, peppers, carrots, beets, cabbage, chard, pumpkin, basil, squash, turnip greens, and dandelion greens. Also include foods with vitamin B such as: liver, oats, tuna, beef, turkey, potatoes, avocados, legumes, brazil nuts, bananas and kefir.

Eat food with whole grain ingredients: Whole grains are high in insoluble fiber; they are complex carbohydrates that have not been processed. They break down slowly releasing continual quantities of glucose into the bloodstream. Whole grains protect you from heart disease, lower risk of breast cancer, boost your immune system and relieve menopausal symptoms. Consume foods that contain whole grain, including: whole grain breads, pastas or brown rice, oats, goats, quinoa and buckwheat grains. Eat about 3 servings a day.

Eat beans more often: Beans are low in fat and high in proteins, they are full of fiber, contain phytoestrogens and help slow the absorption of glucose, keeping you feeling fuller for longer. They also have many minerals and vitamins, including calcium, folic acids and vitamin B6.

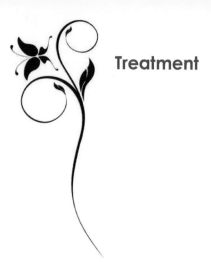

Treatment

Treatment

Sometimes implementing a healthy lifestyle is not easy and some women need to employ a different approach such as alternative medicines and prescriptions drugs.

Alternative Medicines include treatments such as natural herbs, acupuncture, aromatherapy, massage and hypnosis.

Natural remedies or herbs include phytoestrogens and non-estrogenic herbs.

- Phytoestrogens are estrogen like substance found in some plants. There are three types: isoflavones, lignans and coumestans. Isoflavones includes soybeans, chickpeas and legumes. Lignans occur in flaxseeds, wholegrains and some fruit and vegetables. Coumestans include sprouting seeds and alfalfa. Make sure that you eat these foods in moderation as they can also affect your endocrine system and cause tissue growth associated with breast cancer, particularly unfermented soy. They also can affect the natural production of estrogen if you consume then for a long time.
- Non-estrogenic herbs contain no estrogen like substances. These herbs stimulate the body to produce natural hormones in order to reduce postmenopausal symptoms. These herbs have no known side effects. They prevent osteoporosis, protect against cardiovascular disease, improve sexual performance and benefit the endocrine system. The most common non-estrogen herb is "Macafem". Macafem is a perennial plant found in Peru.

Acupuncture involves the stimulation of specific points in the skin either by needles, heat, pressure or laser light.

Aromatherapy uses plant materials, essential oils and other aromatic compounds to alleviate symptoms.

Massage can also alleviate symptoms and reduce stress. Both therapeutic and relaxation massage can be beneficial to treat symptoms.

Hypnosis or hypnotherapy is a method of inducing a deep relaxed state of mind in order to treat disorders or help you to change perceptions or attitudes, such as pain, insomnia, stress, migraines, high blood pressure, etc.

Prescription drugs: includes conventional treatments such as hormonal replacement therapy (HTR).

Hormonal replacement therapy (HTR) can help you to reduce moderate to more severe symptoms. Make sure that you discuss with your doctor all the options, advantages and disadvantages. It is usually recognized as the most effective treatment. This treatment can be used for short period of time (1-5 years), as long term can increase the risk of other health problems.

Some of the risks associated with HTR are: heart disease, blood clots, breast cancer, ovarian cancer, endometrial cancer and gallbladder disease.

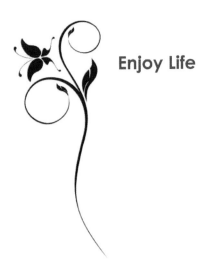

Enjoy Life

Enjoy Life

After going through life, taking care of children and/or family and perhaps building up a career, it is time now to enjoy life.

Spend time doing the things that you love, these can include reading, running, and writing, shopping, or going away with friends.

This can also be a time to try new hobbies or do that "thing" that you always wanted to do, travel, spend more time with your partner or grandchildren or friends. Have fun, have a good laugh, pamper yourself.

Take time to reflect and allow yourself to accept this new phase in your life and   enjoy   it.

Conclusion

Post-menopause is the last stage in women lives. Sometimes women experience depression or anxiety, among many other symptoms associated with hormonal changes in their bodies. Understanding those symptoms can make all the difference in leading a healthy and long life.

It is also a time where women are at risk of contracting serious health diseases. It is important that postmenopausal women have a good understanding of this new phase in their lives and lead healthy lives by having a good diet, exercise and a time to enjoy it.

Reference

www.34-menopause-symptoms.com

www.menopause.org

www.womenhealthpage.com/nutrition

www.womenhealth.com.au

www.betterhealth.vic.gov.au

www.heartfoundation.com.au

www.webmd.com

Thank you

Thank you for reading this book.

I hope you enjoyed it!

If you liked this book I would appreciate if you could take a minute and leave a review with your feedback.

Just go to Amazon.com

Look for **"The Post-menopausal Woman"**

Leading a healthy life.

Living longer.

by Alex Montgomery

and

Click on "write a customer review"

Thank you!

Printed in Great Britain
by Amazon

35725176R00018